The Caregiver's Challenge

The Caregiver's Challenge

John Lowe

Copyright © 2018 by John Lowe.

ISBN:	Hardcover	9781984558497
	Softcover	9781984558480
	eBook	9781984558473

All rights reserved. No part of this book may be reproduced or transmitted in any form or by any means, electronic or mechanical, including photocopying, recording, or by any information storage and retrieval system, without permission in writing from the copyright owner.

The views expressed in this work are solely those of the author and do not necessarily reflect the views of the publisher, and the publisher hereby disclaims any responsibility for them.

Any people depicted in stock imagery provided by Getty Images are models, and such images are being used for illustrative purposes only.
Certain stock imagery © Getty Images.

Print information available on the last page.

Rev. date: 10/08/2018

To order additional copies of this book, contact:
Xlibris
1-888-795-4274
www.Xlibris.com
Orders@Xlibris.com
786432

DEDICATION

This book is dedicated to my wife Connie, without whom this book would never have been written. Connie came into my life having already had two of her nine cancers over her lifetime. As a result of Connie's medical needs throughout our thirty-six years of marriage, I experienced the role of caregiving, and so now it is my hope that I can help those who are willing to take on the role of a caregiver.

I would like to thank all of my children and Christina Aguilar, (my #1 cheerleader, without whose support I truly would have struggled) who supported their mother and friend through all of her cancers and surgeries, especially Mindy, who in the last months of her mother's life, gave up all of her jobs to be there for her mother when I could not.

I would also like to acknowledge all of Connie's friends who provided the much needed support to keep her going, along with all the medical staff who knew and cared for her. I am especially grateful to Dr. Helen Moon, who had the courage to tell Connie that she was finally going to have treatment, both Chemo and radiation to sustain her life. Dr. Moon's decision gave Connie another five plus years of life.

With sincere thanks and gratitude,

John M. Lowe

CONTENTS

Be Supportive 1
Pray 5
Always Work For Tomorrow 7
Be willing to Be Wrong Even If You're Right 9
Share Tears 13
Build a Strong Support Base 17
Accept That Words Are Often Spoken Out of Fear 21
Be Sensitive-You're Not the One Who Is Sick 23
Treat Every Day As Though It Is Your First Day On the Job 27
When the Day Comes, Just Be There to Share 31

Dear Caregiver,

Each of you has taken on one of the hardest jobs in the world, and you are to be commended for that. The pay will not always be what it should be, but in the end, your reward will be the greatest ever. You wil have both good and bad days in your role as a caregiver. Build on the good days and try your best to throw away the bad days. You are a strong and caring person and have accepted a calling which few can fulfill. The challenges you have will be tough, but always remember you are a caregiver because you are tougher than any of these challenges. It is my hope that the few words I share with you in this book will give you the extra strength you will need in your caregiving endeavor. Always strive for the words, "Thank you for a job well done."

Sincerely,

John Michael Lowe

BE SUPPORTIVE

AS I STATED in the foreword, you have taken on one of the hardest jobs as a caregiver. I want to share with you three focal points to focus on as a caregiver. They are to be there for your patient, remain positive, and most importantly, share love.

Generally speaking, there are two reasons that you have chosen to become a caregiver. Either you are a family member or you are trying to earn extra money because you care for people. If you are a family member, your job will be the most challenging because what you have had for so long has changed. Your family member will now need you, and expect things from you instead of being able to do the things they have always done for you. As an outside person of the family, you will also have some challenges, such as getting to know this stranger and to be strong enough to care. If you are a caregiver solely for the extra money, it might be better to find another job because your gain will not come right away.

The first thing you will need to do is to learn how to be there for your patient. If you are a family member, you will soon find out that being there for them now is not the same as before they became ill. Now you must be ready for what was once requested of you to become a demand. You will have to be strong for the patient now, and the best way to overcome this obstacle is to love them even more than you did before they became ill. Now those who have become a caregiver as a job will also have hurdles to overcome, but if you are the person you believe you are, you can do this. Each of you, unlike the family member, are going to be able to start fresh just like making a new friend. You will get the benefits of building a relationship with your patient. Understanding will come to you the more time you spend with him or her, but always remember they need you to be there no matter how hard it is. If and when the day comes that you don't feel you can handle it anymore, take a step back and let someone else take over. Remember, your main priority is always the well being of the patient, and always put them and their needs first. Emotions can deter your ability to carry out the job or responsibility of being a caregiver. Always know that is okay and you did your best.

One of the biggest troubles you will face as a caregiver will be the ability to stay positive. When you first come into the role of caregiving, your patient will still be able to keep a positive attitude, but as the illness progresses, their attitude may revert to negativity as those around them, such as doctors or nurses, begin to speak impersonally about their condition. That is when you will have to encourage a positive outlook in them. Always be there for your patient, and help them know that you, as well as many others, are standing by their side to help them each day. Reinforce their value to others each and every day, and give them a reason to go on living.

The most important part of your role as a caregiver will be to share love with them. Make your patient feel needed, whether it is through words or actions. Family members, this will, more often than not, be easier for you, but you will face some challenges as the illness gets worse. As the illness gets worse, it will be harder on you, so always keep a hug in your arms to wrap around your loved one. Sharing love may many times be the hardest part of your job, depending on how the day went, but always remember it is about the patient and not you. Now, caregivers who come to the patient as a stranger, you will face some challenges also. You, upon arrival to this job, may often be met with belligerent thoughts and words, and maybe even rejection, but, consider the patient's emotions. Answer the patient with a loving heart with the first visit, and as time goes on, you will grow on each other, and you too, will become just like family to him or her.

Finally, always be there even when you don't feel needed because, I can assure you, you are needed. Always promote a positive attitude. You will be faced with a lot of negativity, but be able to counter the negatives with positives. Remember, the thought process begins with what is said and done.

PRAY

YOU, CAREGIVERS, WILL find that the power of prayer is an essential element of caregiving. Never stop believing in the power of prayer because it is a major help in caregiving and helping your patient fight and survive. No matter who it is that you draw your strength from in prayer, use it because it will help you.

By the time you enter your patient's life, there is a good chance they are already praying to the one they believe is going to heal them, so do not worry about using prayer to help. If they pray to a source other than your own, do not discourage it, but remember it is all about your patient and who or what he or she believes will help them heal through this illness. If and when your patient rejects your prayers, as some may do, pray each day when you start the job because you may need it as well depending on the way the day has gone for your patient.

"A Caregiver's Prayer"

Help me today to be the best person, and as helpful as necessary to get my patient through another day. Give me the strength to support my patient, no matter what the day may throw in my direction, be it words or actions. Let me always have an open ear to my patient, the patience to help them, and the understanding of where they are coming from. Make me a source of comfort as they need it each day, and help me to listen to them, knowing when it is best not to say anything. I am here to make my patient's day easier, not my own. With your help, I will be all that I need to be for my patient today. Thank you.

Never force prayer on your patient because their time to pray will come on its own. It will come on its own because at some point, they will feel the need for extra strength, which may not be able to come from you or them. Pray as you need to each day, and the ability to care for your patient will come much easier.

ALWAYS WORK FOR TOMORROW

THE BELIEF IN, and the expectation of tomorrow is possibly your patient's greatest asset, as it very well may be for you also. Someone once said, "Tomorrow never comes," and while this may be true, the ability to focus on the next day will give your patient the desire to go on.

One of the best things you can do as a caregiver for your patient will be to set goals, give your patient something to look forward to. Give them day to day goals, but also, set at least one long range goal. Day to day goals can be as simple as going to the park, or maybe a movie, anything but just sitting at home doing the same old thing. Next, set a long range goal, like someone's graduation or wedding. Remember, you are there to help to help the person you are taking care of to want to live for the next day, or major event.

Always greet your patient each day with a positive thought such as, good morning, how nice to see you this morning. Next, remind them of the plans you made for this day, and as long as they are able, help them fulfill their plans.

At the end of each day, remember that you are always working for tomorrow. Leave your patient with the words, see you in the morning, or see you tomorrow. By using the future tense, you will have implanted in their mind that they will another day, and as a result, they can go to sleep with no cares or worries, and look forward to another day.

BE WILLING TO BE WRONG EVEN IF YOU'RE RIGHT

IN YOUR JOB as a caregiver, you may be faced with many arguments with your patient, most of which may be trivial to you, but to your patient it matters. Always be sure to remind yourself of who is most important during your disagreements. Your job is to relieve the stress rather than creating more during this difficult time for him or her. Three things will be essential in your role as a caregiver. Always know and be mindful of the doctor's plan, make a plan that will help you help achieve that doctor's plan, and last, be willing to be wrong even if you are right.

First in your role as a caregiver, try to share all your patient's doctor visits with them. The reason for this is so both of you will hear the doctor's directions and goals together. Believe me, this is a critical aspect and it will no doubt make your job easier having two pairs of ears instead of just one. Your patient may not always be in the best frame of mind at the doctor's visit, so you are going to be the one that helps the doctor at home. Always remember to take notes because they will be your best defense if your patients begins arguing about what was said during the appointment. Remember, the quicker the argument is resolved, the less stress is created in that moment by your patient and yourself.

Next, prepare your own plan to carry out your patient's doctor's recommendations at home. I would suggest strongly that you start with a daily schedule. Help your patient learn your routine to make your job easier on both of you. Obviously you cannot be too flexible with your patient's medications, but other parts of your routine may be modified depending on what kind of day your patient is having. If it is a day after some form of treatment or therapy, you may expect your patient to be tired or fatigued, as well as somewhat depressed, so try to go with what is best for your patient. If and when you alter their schedule, make sure that your general routine is followed for the most part by the end of the day. Here is an example of a routine I might use:

1. Oral hygiene in the morning
2. Breakfast (essential because most medications will have food requirements) and medication
3. Some form of exercise (a walk or mild stretching depending on your patient)
4. Social time (the meals are a great time)
5. Find an activity your patient enjoys and share it with them, be it reading, games, television, or anything else your patient chooses.

Your key focus points need to be nutrition, medications, exercise, and rest whenever it is needed.

My final point is to be willing to be wrong, even if you are right. If your patient is having a bad day, recognize this. As a caregiver, the first thing you should be doing with your patient is observing their general behavior. This will be instrumental in helping your patient every day, and it will make your job much easier. When you can recognize their bad days, be willing to be wrong if your patient wants you to change your everyday schedule. It will be alright as long as you mind their nutrition, medications, and get out of bed each day. A point that I cannot emphasize enough is that it is your patient's comfort and stress that you are trying to preserve rather than your own. If you begin trying to make it about you, find a new job! If you truly care about your patient, you will be able to find ways to compromise and still fulfill your responsibilities.

If you follow the three basic guidelines I've shared with you, the relationship that you and your patient share will be a lasting one. If conflicts should arise about the doctor's orders, pull out your office visit notes. Next, create your own plan but be flexible according to your patient's needs for the day. Last, be willing to be wrong as long as your patient, as well as the doctor's orders, are followed. If you can follow these guidelines, your role as a caregiver will be one of your most rewarding experiences.

SHARE TEARS

SHARE TEARS, YOU ask? Yes, you must always share tears. Now you may ask why and wonder if there is a reason for this idea. The answer is yes.

I know when I was growing up, I received many spankings from my father, and I still remember the tears I shed and how alone I felt. My siblings would often see me crying after I got punished with a spanking and they would start making fun of me, and it really hurt me that they could not, at the very least, show compassion towards me, even if it was just leaving me alone in my room. Sometimes, the pain of them mocking and ridiculing me was worse than the spanking itself. I tell you this to exemplify how not to act towards a patient.

As a caregiver there will be times of tears for you because of the compassion you build up for your patient. Tears will often come without warning and this is good, especially if you can control them. You may ask why you must control your tears, and for this question, I have two answers. First, you must realize where you are. If you are in the doctor's office with your patient, let your emotions flow with the patient. There is nothing wrong with your tears at this time, in fact, it may strengthen your bond with your patient because it will show how much you really do care. Remember, your actions should always be in your patient's best interest.

A time to try to hold back tears is the time when they are shed for your own personal feelings you may feel on your patient's bad days, or maybe bad days of your own. Emotional stability for the one you are caring for is always first and foremost, and when they are having a bad day, no matter how hard it may be, try to stay strong for your patient.

Think of ways to bring happiness back to them. By now you will know what your patient enjoys and what helps to cheer them up. On your lunch break, go and get them a small gift, whether it's flowers or a small donut, to put a smile on their face again.

On your bad days, which you will have and are entitled to, think about your patient. If there is something in your personal life that you are really struggling with, take the day off. Believe it or not, the patient builds a bond with you, and they will feel your emotions, possibly causing them more stress. This would not be a good situation or environment for your patient, so taking the day off would be beneficial for not only yourself, but your patient as well. They will understand, as they know you need days off, and in doing so, you will be putting your patient first.

For many of you, particularly those of you who are men, you may consider tears to be a sign of weakness because that is, too often, the way we were raised. Believe me, the day will come when the tears are just going to start flowing, especially if it is a family member for which you are caring for. Do not fight your tears, however, because this is your mind and body releasing the tension that has been built up over the situation. It will be at this time that you will realize the importance of tears. When you release that tension with your tears, your "macho" level will be taken down a notch and you will be able to see why it is alright to share your tears with your patient after so long of holding them in.

To conclude, I would just like to tell you that when the day comes that you shed your first real tear, a barrier is broken once and for all. The tears that come to you as a result of punishment, like those I once released as a child, are nothing compared to those that you shed for others in your life. Once you have overcome the belief in your upbringing that crying is a form of weakness, the hardships of life will become much easier to face. The flowing of tears becomes like the cloud that can no longer contain the moisture it holds and releases all of the pressure, as with yourself as a caregiver, opening once more to repeat the cycle. You will always be able to handle all of the hardships with your patient if you keep your emotions healthy as well. Hold your head up high, and shed your tears to make your role as a caregiver much happier.

BUILD A STRONG SUPPORT BASE

AS A CAREGIVER, your focus must be on how both the patient and yourself are going to get through this illness the easiest way possible. The answer to why it is necessary to build a strong support base is not always obvious, but here I will explain mine to you.

First, let me tell you about what I call the obvious support group in every patient's life, the family. As a caregiver, it is reasonable to expect that your patient's family is going to be your strongest ally in this job, however, do not count on them. The family can be going through different stages, including assumptions or rejection. If your patient has had many medical issues in their life, unfortunately, their family may have adapted to believe that their loved one will be just fine, as it has happened in the past. This may or may not be the case whether they know or not, so as the caregiver you can also help them to understand that nothing is guaranteed.

Next, for those caregivers who are not a direct member of the family, you may see that the family may reject the fact that the patient has been diagnosed with more than just a common cold. If one has not experienced the illness themselves, it is hard to put themselves in another's circumstance. If this should happen, never argue with the family about their thoughts because it may be one of the times when you will need to be willing to be wrong in your discussion with the patient's family. You, as a caregiver, will be the most convincing to the family by the actions you show toward your patient. Show the family how much you care for your patient with whatever emotions arise inside you. When the family sees your passion for their loved one, take the time to explain the seriousness of the illness, and as time goes on, the family may get a better understanding of the true situation their loved one faces. After all, they did hire you.

Last, let your patient reach out to any and every source they feel is a strong support base for them. This may be friends, a club, an organization or church. The larger the support base they have, the more fight your patient will have to get through this.

Now I will focus on you as the caregiver. When you took on this role, you became the number one supporter of your patient even, if it is solely because of the amount of time you spend with them. As I stated earlier, this job you filled can and will be one of the hardest tasks of your life both professionally and personally. The obvious will not always be, but you will need their family working alongside you to make your job easier. One of the best things you can do as a caregiver is to become a part of, and relate to, the family, Show them that your patient is not just a job or a paycheck to you, but rather a person you care about as much as they do. Let the family know you are on their side too, after all, you may be listening and hearing the patient's emotions more often than the family does.

The support base in this situation is not only crucial to your patient, but to you as well. You must always take care of yourself in order to be able to take care of anyone else. Unlike your patient, you will generally not be able to turn to your family for support and understanding. There are two reasons for this. The first reason is because of confidentiality purposes. How can you speak to your family about a situation that is not yours to talk about? The second reason is that the emotions you endure throughout the day cannot always be expressed through words hours after you have felt them. They cannot feel an attachment that you have created with your patient and may see this as just another job in your life. You must be able to understand this, but still use your family as much as you can for the support they can give to you. If at all posssible, look for a caregiver's support group because it will be there that you will be able to talk freely about the emotions you are feeling. You will also be able to listen and help your peers that are there sharing their feelings and challenges they are facing, and be surprised to find that many of them are feeling the same way you are some days. Just as your patient has a support base, so should you because you will face bad days as well, though in a different way than your patient.

In closing, let me make suggestions for how you can be the best caregiver for your patient. First, always believe in yourself. Second, always believe in your patient. Third, show caring and compassion for both your patient and their family. Finally, take pride in your role and that this is not just another job, but rather a bond you will have for life. A caregiver is a role few can fill and therefore this should not be taken lightly.

ACCEPT THAT WORDS ARE OFTEN SPOKEN OUT OF FEAR

CAN YOU EVER remember a time when you were so afraid that words would not come out, and even if they did, you did not want to repeat them? We have all been there before, at some point in our lives, and your patient probably will too.

Many times as a caregiver, your patient will have gotten news that has upset them and they start to feel afraid of what's going to happen to them. At this time, you may be the only sounding board they have to vent on. Sometimes their words will hurt, but when you are struggling with your patient's actions, try wearing their shoes for a moment and try to understand why they are reacting the way they are. If you are there for them during the bad news time, your patient will no doubt handle things better and this is the most helpful part of your job. Being able to share their tears and fears without saying a word is the most support you can give to them.

As you, the caregiver, hear the same news your patient has, your compassion will cause you to want to verbalize your frustrations with them because you are human as well. Try to hold onto your emotions, though, in order to better support your patient. There will be times that you just want to yell and release those frustrations and your sadness, but if at all possible, try to do this away from your patient so that they can look to you as a pillar of strength. Words misspoken are rarely accepted well, but there will be situations that you must accept whatever words that your patient speaks from their mouth. At this time, remember, it is best just to lend your ears and refrain from speaking your thoughts as your patient needs to vent and open themselves to you, the one they trust.

Unfortunately, anger and fear many times feed off each other, so as the caregiver, try to dispel the fear that your patient has by creating something to take their mind off off this news, or whatever negativity at this time in their life.

I stated earlier, as I will many times in this book, that you have boldly taken on one of the most difficult jobs there is, but you can handle it with the inner strength that caregivers have. Always see the whole picture behind the words thrown your way, and use your compassionate nature as a caregiver to help your patient and yourself to make everything well. You are above the angry words thrown your way and when you react in a positive way, the family of the patient will also have the confidence to go on. At the end of the day, brush off any angry words spoken in fear, and be content that on this day that you did your best and look forward to what the morning will bring.

BE SENSITIVE-YOU'RE NOT THE ONE WHO IS SICK

AS A CAREGIVER you will no doubt be challenged in many ways by your patient. We discussed one of those ways as the subject of the previous chapter. Now I want to address sensitivity issues. Your patient may ask, "Why does nobody seem to care?", "Who does the doctor think he is saying things like that to me?", "If there is a God, where is He now?", or even say things like "It's no use, I just want to give up.".

One of the toughest things you will have to help your patient through is helping them to understand that people do care. As a caregiver, you are going to hear their question, "Why doesn't anyone care," often, and always remember that is why you have been hired or are taking care of them. The patient can no longer be by themselves safely. At a certain point your patient will begin making everything all about them. This will generally begin when you first start working with your patient because the patient's family and/or friends are unable to be around as much as required to keep the patient safe. You must do your best at all times to bridge this transition with ease and let your patient know, when you first begin, why you are there, whether it is because family cannot be around enough due to work or other factors, or because they don't feel they are qualified enough to take on this task. Not everyone can fill the role of a caregiver, even if they are family of the patient. Always know that when you come into your patient's life, you have just become a part of the family, and your patient may even need you to fill the void the family has involuntarily left by not being around as much. Until you gain their trust, however, the person you are caring for is going to feel abandoned and possibly that nobody cares although you know that they do.

One of the best things that the person you are caring for can do for you is constantly ask you, "Why am I not getting better?" Encourage this process from your patient because by asking this question, they are making a choice for their future and they believe that whatever the doctor is doing for them will make them better. Never take away anything the patient offers that can be made into a positive because when you look for positivity in them and build on it, that is a majority of the battle. Many patients do not hear positive comments each day, but with you there, you can emphasize that there is positivity to this situation even more, whether they can see it or not. Let them know that the healing will take time. The positivity you provide each day can be as simple as "Wow! You walked a long way today!" Anything will make them feel better if they can recognize that you notice, and do in fact care.

Your patient's doctor is always going to play a major role in both your patient and your own life. When it comes to the doctor, look for specific characteristics in them. Will they come down to your level when speaking to your patient or yourself? If you notice that they cannot or will not, find a doctor who can. Communication is key in the healing of a patient because the patient is already vulnerable. Does the doctor show that they care in a way that makes your patient comfortable? To win a battle over an illness, there must be a complete confidence in the doctor giving recommendations and facts regarding that illness.

When you take on the role of caregiving, another question you will hear often is "If there is a God, where is He now?" This is, once again, a big step in the right direction for your patient because they have just told you that they believe, or at least have faith in a higher power. This will be a huge help in your caregiving. Encourage your patient that sometimes they are being used to bring an example to others, and by sharing this thought, your patient may feel that they have a purpose. As a caregiver, you want to seize any opportunity to build your hope in your patient. Keep your patient focused on what their thought of their higher power can do for them, especially when they begin to think that they have been completely abandoned by their source of strength.

The hardest thing you may have to deal with will be when your patient gets to the point of giving up. This will come when your patient has gone through all the steps we have focused on in this chapter. Now is the time that you must be the most sensitive to your patient. If and when you reach this point in your role as a caregiver, just be quiet and listen. They will have a lifetime of stories to share with you, and each day that you are willing to just listen is one more day your patient has given themselves. At the end of each day, ask to hear more stories the next day. By doing this, you will not only learn more from and about your patient, but also make them happier and their thoughts of giving up may be extinguished, even if it's for just a moment. You may hear the same stories repeatedly, but keep in mind that if they feel the need to repeat them, the stories probably mean the most and will help the most.

I would like to encourage you to make a special time each week, probably when the fewest people involved in your patient's life are working, to get the family together to listen to your patient's stories. Do not put a time frame on this activity because this time is for your patient. When you are able to do this, everything that has been discussed in this chapter will become more bearable for your patient. By setting aside this time, your patient will feel a sense of purpose, and their family will get to hear more about them, as you did, and will cherish it for a lifetime. Be sensitive, and never forget, you are not the one who is sick, so be there for your patient as much as possible.

TREAT EVERY DAY AS THOUGH IT IS YOUR FIRST DAY ON THE JOB

ALTHOUGH I KEEP emphasizing this point, as a caregiver you have taken on one of the most difficult roles in the world. Your career is going to have many ups and downs, so it will be important to reflect on why you decided on this career. If the day ever comes when you don't feel the way you did on the first day of your job, it may be a wise decision to leave this career and find another one. As you read this, you may wonder if that is a bit harsh or a rather dramatic decision, but I will explain why.

One of the first reasons you may leave this career is because you struggle with all of the ups and downs that come with it. Fortunately, you may be able to realize this early on in the career. Many times, caregivers are belittled by their patients because they have so many people speaking to them as though they are a child, or as though they have no idea what is going on. As a result, all of the compassion you had for this career may fade because you hadn't realized what is unacceptable in other careers is, not necessarily acceptable in caregiving, but definitely understandable and expected. Hopefully, if you begin feeling this way, you remove yourself from this position quickly because neither your patient nor yourself will benefit from the feelings you gain from this experience. If you do decide to leave this career, never hang your head in shame or feel less of a person. Instead, be happy that you tried, and realized that it was not the career for you. You will be opening the door to someone who may be better suited to care for your patient, and in doing so, still putting your patient's best interest first. Always remember, it takes a bigger person to walk away from this career than to stay with it, knowing they would not be fulfilling the caregiver's role properly, for a paycheck.

Next, there will be those of you who truly are called to be a caregiver, those who are the strongest of the strong, and you are able to face any challenge your patient throws your way. You are a real caregiver. You will have the ability to make the positives in your career outweigh the negatives, a task very few are able to accomplish in this circumstance. You will always be able to uplift the spirits of the one you are caring for because you have been chosen to give the gift of caregiving. After a bad day the patient had previously, you will be abe to come back the next day with a positive attitude, a smile on your face, and act as though it is the first day on the job. On this day, your patient will see the joy you receive from caring for them and that negativity of the day before will be disspelled. Once again, your role as a true caregiver will be reinforced. You will know that you were chosen for this role and will display this, not only for your patient and yourself, but also for their family and friends. You will truly be one of those who are chosen for this very precious role and, believe me, you will be noticed and appreciated.

Another type of caregiver is the one who shows compassion for their patient. Those are most often the family members who want to see their loved one as happy as they have been thorughout their life. I want to warn you, however, that if you are that family member caregiver, you must be willing to push your family member out of their comfort zone because, if you don't, they can deteriorate very fast. The last thing you want your patient to do is make decisions in matters regarding their improvement, such as medications, nutrition, exercise, and environment. Your loved one and you know what the doctor ordered. If a doctor orders a specific diet that your loved one may not want to follow, try to vary it to your patient's desire, but only in ways that are equally as beneficial as the doctor's suggestions. In any matter, however, you must not back down to your loved one if they disagree. Even if they cannot see it, you are doing what is best for them. When it comes to the doctor's orders about exercise, make the exercise as fun and adventurous as possible. Make it something that your patient wants to do, rather than has to do. As a family member, your role as a caregiver will be the most difficult, and if you can do it successfully, I give you all commendment in the world because I know, through my experience, what you have to endure from the rewards to the sacrifices.

In closing, I want to reiterate the importance of treating each day as if it were your first day on the job. I've spoken on a few different scenarios of caregivers, and, don't get me wrong, whether you only lasted a day or two or you lasted many years as a caregiver, each of you are to be commended. Each day you woke up, you were able to treat it as your first day on the job, and when you could not do this anymore, you ultimately thought about your patient and what was best for them, passing on the reigns to someone else no matter how much it hurt. As with anything in life, there are those who have the true calling to a profession, and those who just want to be there to help. No matter what the case may be, each of you will have done your best, and your patient will always be better for what you have done. Stand tall, and always hold your head up high!

WHEN THE DAY COMES, JUST BE THERE TO SHARE

YOU, AS A caregiver, will always know that the next day is never promised or guaranteed, and this is what makes you a special person not only to your patient, but also to your patient's family. Whether it is during the healing process, or the unfortunate end of your patient's life, you will be so important and I will tell you why.

As a caregiver you most likely will be more like family to them than your patient's own family. While this is not the way it should be, in reality, this is the way it usually turns out. When you first take on this role, the family members are going to want to be there nonstop, but as the days go on and your patient weakens, able to do less than before, the family often begins being around less and less no matter how much you may encourage them to be around more often. You will, as a caregiver, have the insight to understand where the family is coming from. Never demean the family for their actions, but instead put yourself in their shoes once in a while. This will help you understand what they are going through. They are seeing their once active and energetic family member now becoming unable to do much on their own. Do not pity the family, but have compassion for them instead during this challenging time.

Your role as a caregiver, although difficult, will be the most rewarding if you choose to listen more than to speak. As the time gets closer to your patient's final goodbye, they may want to take you on their life journey. They will speak mostly of the highlights of their life, and sometimes about the most sensitive things that have happened in their life, and this is why you must always be willing to listen. Remember when I stated before that as the time with your patient goes on, you will ultimately become like their closest family member as they share their deepest and closest memories.

You, as the caregiver, are going to hold the key to the family's ultimate closure of your patient's life. This is because you had the insight to take the time to listen. Sure, in your mind at the time, you were just occupying time, but now that your patient has passed, do not hold your patient's words inside. Share them with the family. You often enjoyed their stories, and although they may have even bored you if they were repeated over over, you now have the opportunity to give the family a gift of a lifetime. Since you took the time to listen when family members could not, you will now be able to share this most valuable gift, your patient's stories, as only your patient could tell them. Once you've passed their stories on, you will finally be paid in full. Not paid in dollars and cents of course, but with love from one who, at the beginning may have been a complete stranger, but became like your own family. As I close this Caregiver's Handbook, all I can say to you, as the caregiver, is "Thank you for a job well done."

www.ingramcontent.com/pod-product-compliance
Lightning Source LLC
Chambersburg PA
CBHW031554210526
45464CB00003B/1298